Sweet Dash Diet Slow Cooker Meals

50 Different Recipes for your Sweet Moments

Carmela Rojas

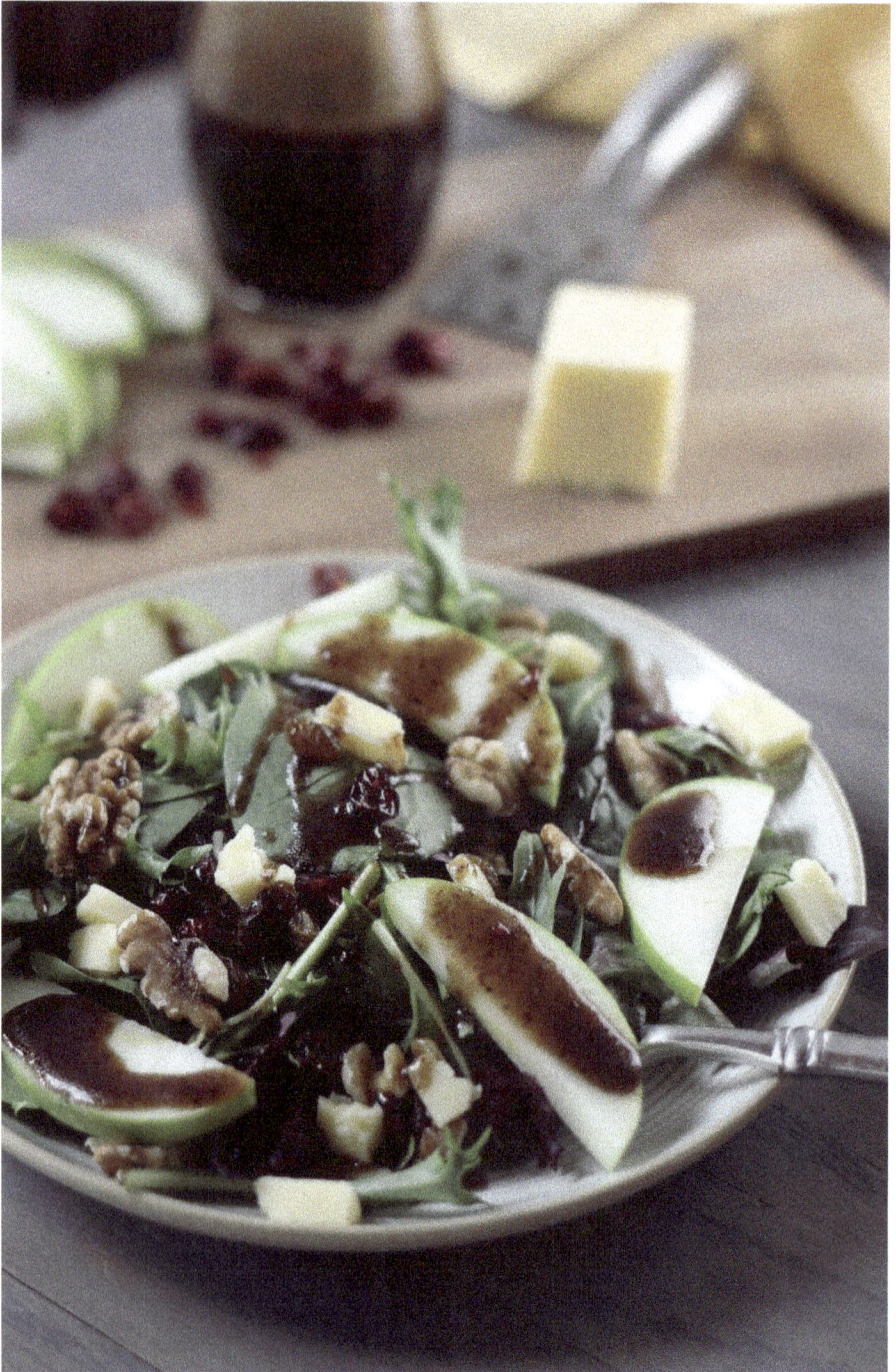

indirect, which are incurred as a result of the use of information contained within this document, including, but not limited to, — errors, omissions, or inaccuracies.

Table of Contents

Cored Apples with Raisins

Servings: 4

Cooking Time: 4 Hours

Ingredients:

- A handful raisins
- 4 big apples, cored and cut into wedges
- 2 tablespoons natural apple juice
- 2 tablespoons stevia
- 1 tablespoon cinnamon powder

Directions:

1. In your slow cooker, mix the apples with the raisins, cinnamon, apple juice and stevia, cover and cook on Low for 4 hours.
2. Divide into bowls and serve warm.

Nutrition Info:

Calories 151, Fat 1.9g, Cholesterol 0mg, Sodium 17mg, Carbohydrate 40.9g, Fiber 6g, Sugars 25.5g, Protein 1.1g, Potassium 242mg

Pumpkin Puree Dip

Servings: 8

Cooking Time: 8 Hours

Ingredients:

- 1 cup pumpkin puree
- 8 apples, cored, peeled and sliced
- 1/3 cup water
- 1/3 cup palm sugar
- ½ teaspoon pumpkin pie spice
- ¼ teaspoon nutmeg, ground

Directions:

1. In your slow cooker, combine the apples with the sugar, pumpkin puree, water, spice and nutmeg, stir, cover and cook on Low for 8 hours.

2. Blend using an immersion blender, divide into bowls and serve as a sweet dip.

9

Nutrition Info:

Calories 167, Fat 0.5g, Cholesterol 0mg, Sodium 491mg, Carbohydrate 43.4g, Fiber 6.3g, Sugars 33.g, Protein 1g, Potassium 713mg

Maple Syrup Poached Pears

Servings: 4

Cooking Time: 4 Hours

Ingredients:

- 2 cups grapefruit juice
- 4 pears, peeled and cored
- ¼ cup maple syrup
- 1 tablespoon ginger, grated
- 2 teaspoons cinnamon powder

Directions:

1. In your slow cooker, mix pears with grapefruit juice, maple syrup, cinnamon and ginger, cover, cook on Low for 4 hours, divide everything into bowls and serve.

Nutrition Info:

Calories 214, Fat 0.5g, Cholesterol 0mg, Sodium 5mg, Carbohydrate 55.3g, Fiber 7.9g, Sugars 40.2g, Protein 1.6g, Potassium 461mg

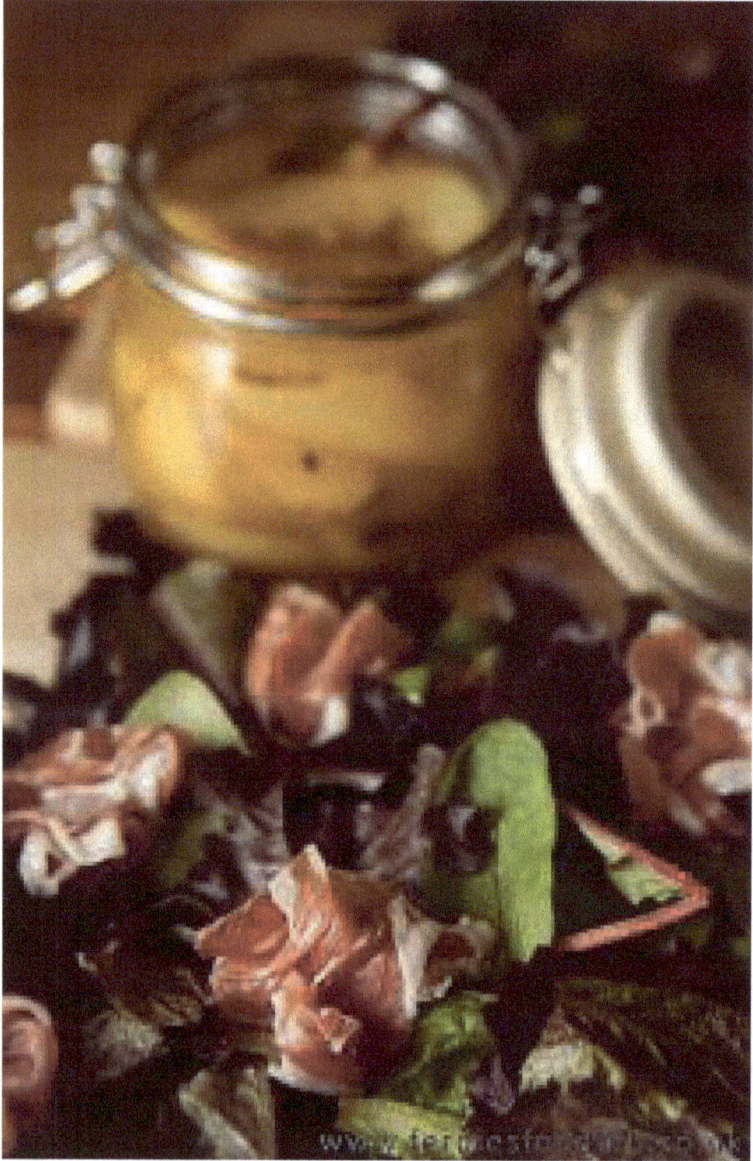

Almond Quinoa

Servings: 4

Cooking Time: 4 Hours

Ingredients:

- 1 teaspoon vanilla extract
- 1 cup quinoa
- 1/8 coconut flakes
- ¼ cup cranberries
- 2 teaspoons stevia
- 3 cups coconut water
- 1/8 cup almonds, sliced

Directions:

1. In your slow cooker, mix the coconut water with the quinoa, vanilla, stevia, coconut, almonds and cranberries, cover and cook on Low for 4 hours.
2. Stir the quinoa mix, divide it between plates and serve for breakfast.

Nutrition Info:

Calories 259, Fat .8.6g, Cholesterol 0mg, Sodium 194mg, Carbohydrate 39.3g, Fiber 6.7g, Sugars 6g, Protein 8.4g, Potassium 768mg

Chocolate Bars

Servings: 12

Cooking Time: 2 Hours And 30 Minutes

Ingredients:

- 1 cup coconut sugar
- ½ cup dark chocolate chips
- 1 egg white
- ¼ cup coconut oil, melted
- ½ teaspoon vanilla extract
- 1 teaspoon baking powder
- 1 and ½ cups almond meal

Directions:

1. In a bowl, mix the oil with sugar, vanilla extract, egg white, baking powder and almond flour and whisk well
2. Fold in chocolate chips and stir gently.
3. Line your slow cooker with parchment paper, grease it, add cookie mix, press on the bottom, cover and cook on low for 2 hours and 30 minutes.
4. Take cookie sheet out of the slow cooker, cut into medium bars and serve.

Nutrition Info:

Calories 141, Fat 11.8g, Cholesterol 0mg, Sodium 7mg, Carbohydrate 7.7g, Fiber 1.5g, Sugars 3.2g, Protein 3.2g, Potassium 134mg

Hot Fondue

Servings: 8

Cooking Time: 1 Hr

Ingredients:

- ¼ Corn Syrup (light)
- ½ cup Soy Milk
- ½ cup Margarine (vegan)
- ½ tbsp. Vanilla Extract
- 8 oz. Chocolate Chips (semisweet and dark)
- Salt

Directions:

1. Place all the ingredients except Vanilla and chocolate chips in the slow cooker.
2. Cook on "low" for 1 hr.
3. Stir once and again cook for another hr on "low".Add in rest of the ingredients. Mix well so that chocolate will melt thoroughly.
4. Serve with fruit.

Nutrition Info:

(Estimated Amount Per Serving): 318 Calories; 25 g Total Fats; 16 mg Sodium; 0 mg Cholesterol; 26 g Carbohydrates; 1.5 g Dietary Fiber; 1.5 g Protein

Orange Juice Dip

Servings: 4

Cooking Time: 2 Hours And 30 Minutes

Ingredients:

- 12 ounces cranberries
- 1 cup coconut sugar
- 2 and ½ teaspoons orange zest, grated
- ¼ cup orange juice
- 2 tablespoons maple syrup

Directions:

1. In your slow cooker, mix orange juice with maple syrup, orange zest, sugar and cranberries, stir, cover and cook on High for 2 hours and 30 minutes.

2. Blend using an immersion blender, divide into bowls and serve.

Nutrition Info:

Calories 35, Fat 0g, Cholesterol 0mg, Sodium 4mg, Carbohydrate 7g, Fiber 1.1g, Sugars 3.4g, Protein 0.1g, Potassium 66mg

Tofu Frittata

Servings: 4

Cooking Time: 6 Hours

Ingredients:

- 3 tablespoons garlic, minced
- 1 red bell pepper, chopped
- 1 pound firm tofu, drained, pressed and crumbled
- 2 tablespoons olive oil
- 1 yellow onion, chopped
- ¼ teaspoon turmeric powder
- 1 teaspoon basil, dried
- 1 teaspoon oregano, dried
- 1 tablespoon lemon juice
- ½ cup kalamata olives, pitted and halved
- Black pepper to the taste

Directions:

1. Add the oil to your slow cooker and spread the crumbled tofu.
2. Add onion, turmeric, garlic, bell pepper, olives, basil, oregano, lemon juice and pepper, toss a bit, cover and cook on Low for 6 hours.

3. Divide frittata between plates and serve for breakfast.

Nutrition Info:

Calories 224, Fat 15.2g, Cholesterol 0mg, Sodium 444mg, Carbohydrate 14.5g, Fiber 3g, Sugars 5.8g, Protein 10.8g, Potassium 306mg

Tapioca

Servings: 10 Servings

Ingredients:

- 8 cups (1.9 L) skim milk
- 1¼ cups (250 g) sugar
- 1 cup (125 g) tapioca
- 1 cup (120 ml) egg substitute
- 1 teaspoon vanilla

Directions:

1. Combine milk and sugar in slow cooker, stirring until sugar is dissolved as well as possible. Stir in tapioca. Cover and cook on high 3 hours. In a small mixing bowl, beat egg substitute slightly. Beat in vanilla and about 1 cup (235 ml) hot milk from slow cooker. When well mixed, stir egg mixture into slow cooker. Cover and cook on high 20 more minutes. Chill for several hours. Serve with whipped topping if you wish.

Nutrition Info:

Per serving: 199 g water; 255 calories (5% from fat, 17% from protein, 78% from carb); 11 g protein; 1 g total fat; 0 g saturated

fat; 0 g monounsaturated fat; 0 g polyunsaturated fat; 50 g carb; 0 g fiber; 26 g sugar; 252 mg phosphorus; 298 mg calcium; 1 mg iron; 161 mg sodium; 444 mg potassium; 490 IU vitamin A; 120 mg ATE vitamin E; 2 mg vitamin C; 4 mg cholesterol

Fruit Oats

Servings: 4

Cooking Time: 3 Hours

Ingredients:

- 1 mango, peeled and cubed
- 2 cups non-fat milk
- 1 cup old-fashioned oats
- ½ teaspoon almond extract
- ½ tablespoon sugar

Directions:

1. In your slow cooker, combine the oats with the milk and the other ingredients, toss, put the lid on and cook on High for 3 hours.
2. Divide into bowls into bowls and serve for breakfast.

Nutrition Info:

Calories 178, Fat .1.6g, Cholesterol 2mg, Sodium 67mg, Carbohydrate 33.7g, Fiber 3.3g, Sugars 19.2g, Protein 7.3g, Potassium 404mg

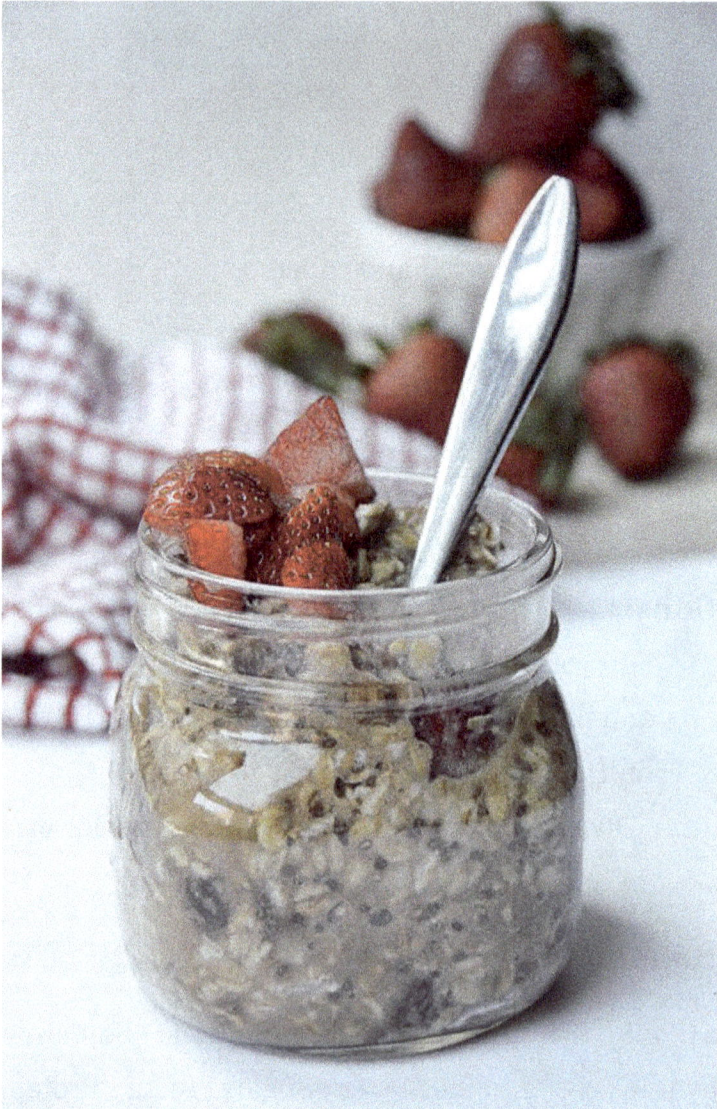

Grapefruit Mix

Servings: 4

Cooking Time: 2 Hours

Ingredients:

- 1 cup water
- 1 cup palm sugar
- 64 ounces red grapefruit juice
- 2 cups grapefruit, peeled and cubed
- ½ cup mint, chopped

Directions:

1. In your slow cooker, mix the water with your grapefruit, sugar, mint and grapefruit juice, stir, cover and cook on High for 2 hours.
2. Divide into bowls and serve cold.

Nutrition Info:

Calories 554, Fat 0.3g, Cholesterol 0mg, Sodium 3122mg, Carbohydrate 139g, Fiber 2.1g, Sugars 67.4g, Protein 1.3g, Potassium 2775mg

Applesauce and Carrot Mix

Servings: 10

Cooking Time: 6 Hours

Ingredients:

- 2 tablespoons stevia
- 1 cup raisins
- 6 cups water
- 2 tablespoons cinnamon powder
- 14 ounces carrots, shredded
- 8 ounces canned pineapple, crushed
- 23 ounces natural applesauce
- 1 tablespoon pumpkin pie spice

Directions:

1. In your slow cooker, mix carrots with applesauce, raisins, stevia, cinnamon, pineapple and pumpkin pie spice, stir, cover, cook on Low for 6 hours, divide into bowls and serve for breakfast.

Nutrition Info:

Calories 110, Fat 0.2g, Cholesterol 0mg, Sodium 42mg, Carbohydrate 29.6g, Fiber 3g, Sugars 19.6g, Protein 0.9g, Potassium 265mg

Berry Yogurt

Servings: About 3

Cooking Time: 1 Hr

Ingredients:

- ¾ cup Blueberries
- ¾ cup Strawberries (chopped)
- ¾ cup Raspberries
- ¾ tsp. Lemon Zest (grated)
- ¾ tsp. Orange Zest (grated)
- ¾ tbsp. Balsamic Vinegar
- Juice ¼ Orange
- 1 ½ cup Greek Yogurt (low fat)
- ¼ tsp. Vanilla Extract
- 3 tbsp. sliced Almonds (toasted)
- Black Pepper (cracked)

Directions:

1. Place all the ingredients except yogurt and almonds in the slow cooker.
2. Cook on "low" for 1 hr.
3. Mash the berries.
4. Divide the yogurt in bowls.

5. Garnish with berry sauce and almonds.

6. Serve.

Nutrition Info:

(Estimated Amount Per Serving): 163 Calories; 4 g Total Fats; 47 mg Sodium; 5 mg Cholesterol; 20 g Carbohydrates; 5 g Dietary Fiber; 14 g Protein

Soft Pudding

Servings: 4

Cooking Time: 1 Hour

Ingredients:

- ½ cup coconut water
- 2 teaspoons lime zest, grated
- 2 tablespoons green tea powder
- 1 and ½cup avocado, pitted, peeled and chopped
- 1 tablespoon stevia

Directions:

1. In your slow cooker, mix coconut water with avocado, green tea powder, lime zest and stevia, stir, cover, cook on Low for 1 hour, divide into bowls and serve.

Nutrition Info:

Calories 120, Fat 10.7g, Cholesterol 0mg, Sodium 35mg, Carbohydrate 8.5g, Fiber 4.4g, Sugars 1.1g, Protein 1.5g, Potassium 362mg

Banana Cream

Servings: 4

Cooking Time: 1 Hour

Ingredients:

- 1 and ½ cup coconut cream
- 2 cups banana, peeled and mashed
- 2 tablespoons maple syrup
- 2 teaspoons lime zest, grated
- 1 tablespoon lime juice

Directions:

1. In your slow cooker, combine the banana with the cream and the other ingredients, put the lid on and cook on High for 1 hour.
2. Divide into bowls and serve cold.

Nutrition Info:

Calories 302, Fat 21.7g, Cholesterol 0mg, Sodium 15mg, Carbohydrate 29.4g, Fiber 4.1g, Sugars 18.3g, Protein 2.9g, Potassium 533mg

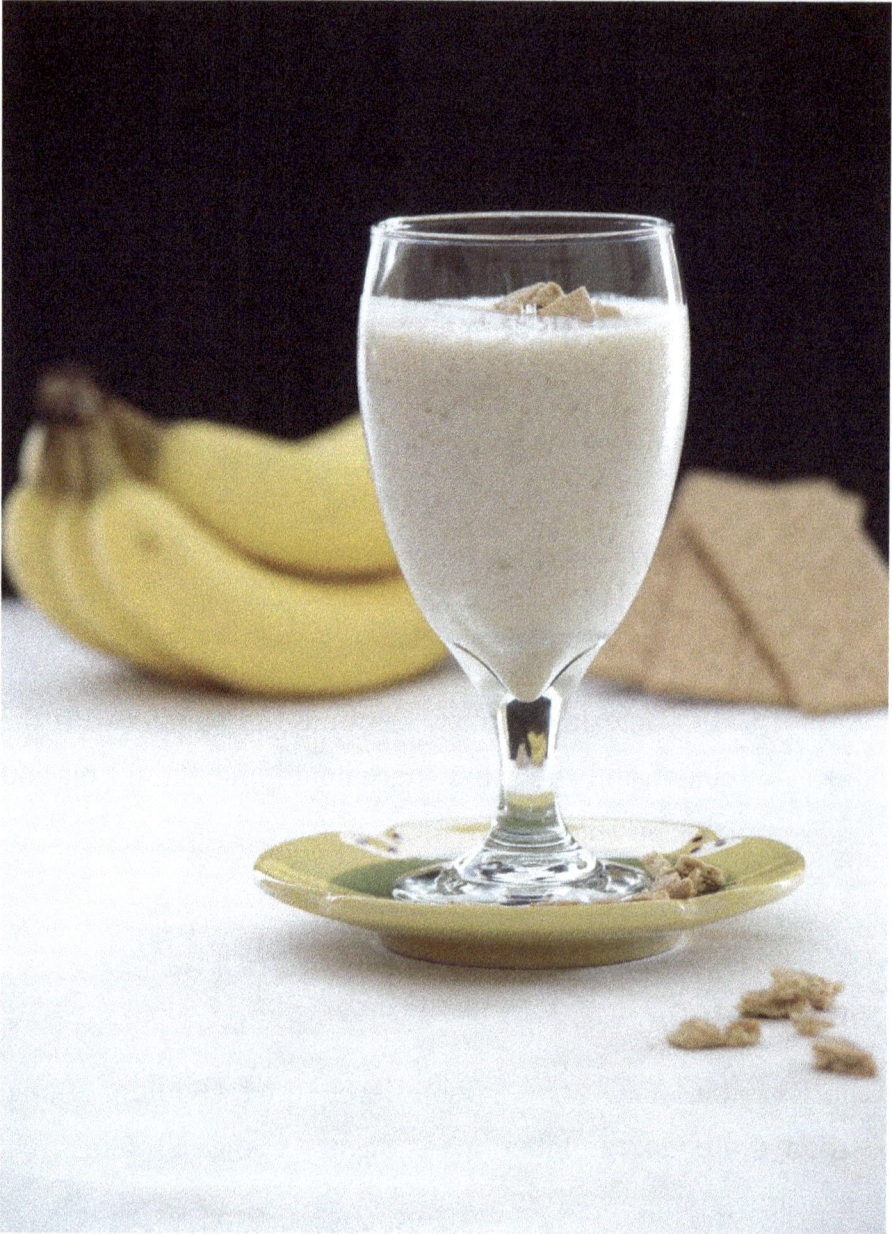

Black Beans Salad

Servings: 4

Cooking Time: 4 Hours

Ingredients:
- 8 eggs, whisked
- 4 spring onions, chopped
- 1 teaspoon chili powder
- ½ teaspoon smoked paprika
- ½ cup low-sodium veggie stock
- A pinch of black pepper
- 1 cup kalamata olives, pitted and halved
- 1 and ½ cups canned black beans, no-salt-added, drained and rinsed

Directions:
1. In the slow cooker, combine the eggs with the spring onions, black beans and the other ingredients, toss, put the lid on and cook on Low for 4 hours.
2. Divide the mix into bowls and serve for breakfast.

Nutrition Info:

Calories 422, Fat .13.5g, Cholesterol 327mg, Sodium 446mg, Carbohydrate 50g, Fiber 12.9g, Sugars 2.8g, Protein 27.5g, Potassium 1260mg

Carrot Pudding

Servings: 8 Servings

Ingredients:

- 1¼ cups (156 g) flour
- 1 teaspoon baking powder
- ½ teaspoon baking soda
- ½ teaspoon cinnamon
- ½ teaspoon ground nutmeg
- ½ cup (120 ml) egg substitute
- ¾ cup (170 g) packed brown sugar
- ½ cup (112 g) unsalted butter
- 1 cup (130 g) sliced carrots
- 1 apple, peeled, cored, and cut in eighths
- 1 medium potato, peeled and cut in pieces
- ¾ cup (110 g) raisins

Directions:

1. Stir together flour, baking powder, baking soda, cinnamon, and nutmeg. Place egg substitute, brown sugar, and butter in blender. Cover and blend until smooth. Add carrot to blender mixture; blend until chopped. Add apple; blend until chopped. Add potato;

blend until finely chopped. Stir carrot mixture and raisins into dry ingredients; mix well. Turn into greased and floured 6-cup (4 L) mold; cover tightly with foil. Place in slow cooker. Cover and cook on high for 4 hours. Remove from cooker. Cool 10 minutes; unmold.

Nutrition Info:

Per serving: 77 g water; 359 calories (30% from fat, 6% from protein, 64% from carb); 6 g protein; 12 g total fat; 7 g saturated fat; 3 g monounsaturated fat; 1 g polyunsaturated fat; 59 g carb; 3 g fiber; 32 g sugar; 111 mg phosphorus; 85 mg calcium; 2 mg iron; 116 mg sodium; 534 mg potassium; 3111 IU vitamin A; 95 mg ATE vitamin E; 7 mg vitamin C; 31 mg cholesterol

Apple Cake

Servings: 8 Servings

Ingredients:

- 1 cup (125 g) flour
- ¾ cup (150 g) sugar
- 2 teaspoons baking powder
- 1 teaspoon cinnamon
- 4 apples, chopped
- ¼ cup (60 ml) egg substitute
- 2 teaspoons vanilla

Directions:

1. Combine flour, sugar, baking powder, and cinnamon. Add apples, stirring lightly to coat. Combine egg substitute and vanilla. Add to apple mixture. Stir until just moistened. Spoon into lightly greased slow cooker. Cover and bake on high 2½ to 3 hours. Serve warm.

Nutrition Info:

Per serving: 64 g water; 172 calories (3% from fat, 6% from protein, 91% from carb); 3 g protein; 1 g total fat; 0 g saturated

fat; 0 g monounsaturated fat; 0 g polyunsaturated fat; 40 g carb; 1 g fiber; 26 g sugar; 59 mg phosphorus; 81 mg calcium; 1 mg iron; 136 mg sodium; 104 mg potassium; 53 IU vitamin A; 0 mg ATE vitamin E; 3 mg vitamin C; 0 mg cholesterol

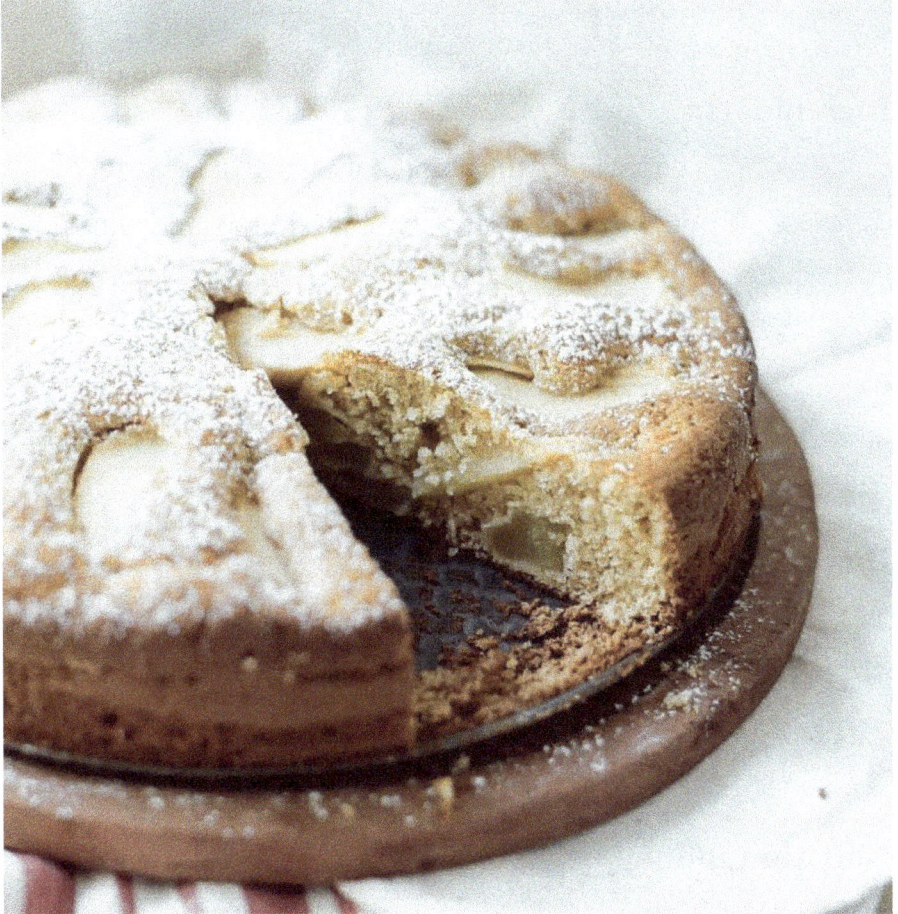

Almond Milk Barley Cereals

Servings: 6

Cooking Time: 6 Hours

Ingredients:

- ½ cup whole wheat and barley cereals
- 4 cups mixed orange, apple, grapes and pineapple pieces
- 12 ounces almond milk
- 2 tablespoons stevia
- ¼ cup coconut, toasted and shredded

Directions:

1. In your slow cooker, mix the fruits with the stevia, cereals and milk, cover and cook on Low for 6 hours.
2. Divide into bowls, sprinkle coconut on top and serve.

Nutrition Info:

Calories 228, Fat 14.9g, Cholesterol 0mg, Sodium 56mg, Carbohydrate 30.8g, Fiber 6g, Sugars 13.3g, Protein 2.6g, Potassium 195mg

Dark Cherry and Stevia Compote

Servings: 6

Cooking Time: 2 Hours

Ingredients:

- 1 pound dark cherries, pitted and halved
- ¾ cup red grape juice
- ¼ cup maple syrup
- ½ cup dark cocoa powder
- 2 tablespoons stevia
- 2 cups water

Directions:

1. In your slow cooker, mix cocoa powder with grape juice, maple syrup, cherries, water and stevia, stir, cover, cook on High for 2 hours, divide into bowls and serve cold.

Nutrition Info:

Calories 132, Fat 1.4g, Cholesterol 0mg, Sodium 179mg, Carbohydrate 37.9g, Fiber 7g, Sugars 23g, Protein 3.2g, Potassium 28mg

Soft Avocado Cream

Servings: 4

Cooking Time: 2 Hours

Ingredients:

- 1 cup avocado, peeled, pitted and mashed
- 2 tablespoons coconut sugar
- 1 cup pumpkin puree
- 1 teaspoon vanilla extract
- 1 teaspoon pumpkin pie spice

Directions:

1. In your slow cooker, combine the avocado with the pumpkin purée and the other ingredients, put the lid on and cook on High for 2 hours.
2. Stir, divide into bowls and serve warm.

Nutrition Info:

Calories 147, Fat 7.3g, Cholesterol 0mg, Sodium 26mg, Carbohydrate 18g, Fiber 4.3g, Sugars 2.4g, Protein 1.9g, Potassium 308mg

Cashews Cake

Servings: 6

Cooking Time: 2 Hours And 30 Minutes

Ingredients:

- 1 and ½ cups avocado, peeled, pitted and mashed
- ½ cup coconut milk
- ½ cup coconut cream
- ½ teaspoon vanilla extract
- 1 cup cashews, chopped
- 4 tablespoons avocado oil
- Juice of 2 limes
- 2 tablespoons coconut sugar

Directions:

1. In your food processor, combine the avocado with the cream and the other ingredients and pulse well.
2. Pour this into the slow cooker lined with parchment paper and cook on High for 2 hours and 30 minutes.
3. Slice and serve cold.

Nutrition Info:

Calories 250, Fat 19.1g, Cholesterol 0mg, Sodium 16mg, Carbohydrate 22.4g, Fiber 4.4g, Sugars 14.4g, Protein 2g, Potassium 390mg

Artichoke Frittata

Servings: 4

Cooking Time: 4 Hours

Ingredients:

- 8 cherry tomatoes, halved
- 1 tablespoon parsley, chopped
- 4 ounces shrimp, peeled, deveined and cut into halves horizontally
- A pinch of black pepper
- A pinch of garlic powder
- 2 eggs
- 4 ounces canned artichokes, drained and chopped
- ¼ cup fat-free milk
- ¼ cup green onions, chopped
- Cooking spray
- 3 tablespoons low-fat cheddar cheese, grated

Directions:

1. In a bowl, mix the eggs with milk, black pepper, garlic powder and green onions and stir well.

2. Grease your slow cooker with the cooking spray, add eggs mix, cover and cook on Low for 3 hours and 30 minutes.

3. Add shrimp, artichokes, cheddar cheese, tomatoes and parsley on top, cover and cook on Low for 30 minutes.

4. Divide frittata between plates and serve for breakfast.

Nutrition Info:

Calories 154, Fat 5.1g, Cholesterol 147mg, Sodium 181mg, Carbohydrate 14.6g, Fiber 4.7g, Sugars 7.9g, Protein 14.3g, Potassium 818mg

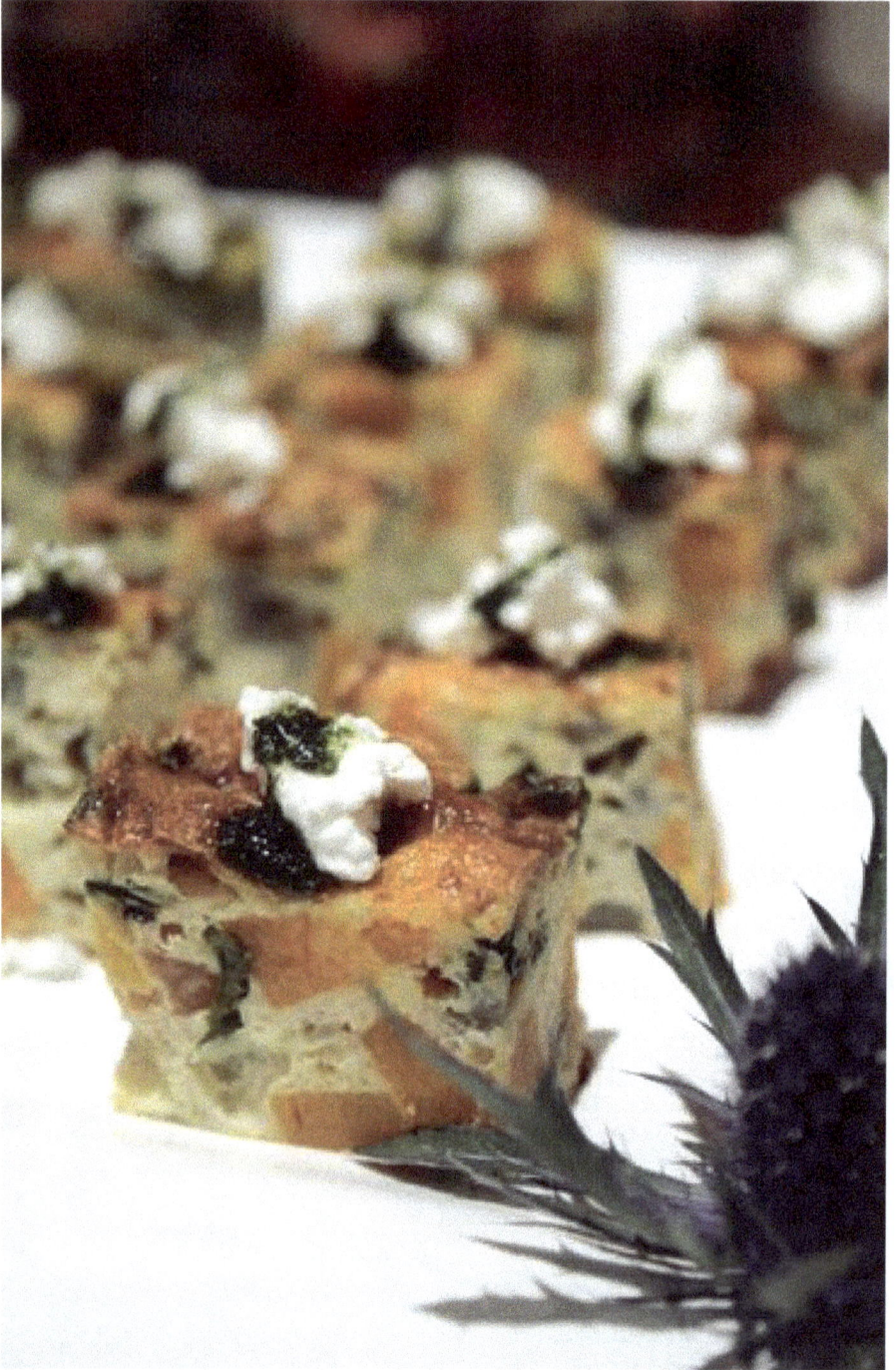

Mexican Eggs

Servings: 8

Cooking Time: 2 Hours

Ingredients:

- 12 ounces low-fat cheese, shredded
- 1 garlic clove, minced
- 1 cup nonfat sour cream
- 10 eggs
- Olive oil cooking spray
- 5 ounces canned green chilies, drained
- 10 ounces tomato sauce, sodium-free
- ½ teaspoon chili powder
- Black pepper to the taste

Directions:

1. In a bowl, mix the eggs with the cheese, sour cream, chili powder, black pepper, garlic, green chilies and tomato sauce, whisk, pour into your slow cooker after you've greased it with cooking oil, cover and cook on Low for 2 hours.
2. Divide between plates and serve.

Nutrition Info: Calories 395, Fat .27.5g, Cholesterol 262mg, Sodium 700mg, Carbohydrate 18.8g, Fiber 5.8g, Sugars 10.6g, Protein 20.9g, Potassium 610mg

Stewed Peach

Servings: 6

Cooking Time: 1 Hour And 30 Minutes

Ingredients:

- 4 cups peaches, cored and roughly chopped
- 4 tablespoons palm sugar
- 2 teaspoons lemon zest, grated
- 6 tablespoons natural apple juice

Directions:

1. In your slow cooker, mix peaches with sugar, apple juice and lemon zest, stir, cover, cook on High for 1 hour and 30 minutes, divide into bowls and serve cold.

Nutrition Info:

Calories 71, Fat 0.3g, Cholesterol 0mg, Sodium 325mg, Carbohydrate 17.3g, Fiber 1.7g, Sugars 16.7g, Protein 1g, Potassium 473mg

Fruited Tapioca

Servings: 6 Servings

Ingredients:

- 2¼ cups (535 ml) water

- 2½ cups (570 ml) pineapple juice

- ½ cup (63 g) tapioca pudding mix

- 1 cup (200 g) sugar

- 15 ounces (420 g) crushed pineapple, undrained

Directions:

1. Mix first four ingredients together in slow cooker. Cover and cook on high 3 hours. Stir in crushed pineapple. Chill for several hours.

Nutrition Info:

Per serving: 241 g water; 267 calories (1% from fat, 1% from protein, 98% from carb); 1 g protein; 0 g total fat; 0 g saturated

fat; 0 g monounsaturated fat; 0 g polyunsaturated fat; 68 g carb;

1 g fiber; 53 g sugar; 14 mg phosphorus; 29 mg calcium; 1 mg iron;

6 mg sodium; 213 mg potassium; 32 IU vitamin A; 0 mg ATE

vitamin E; 16 mg vitamin C; 0 mg cholesterol

Black Pepper Egg Mix

Servings: 4

Cooking Time: 2 Hours

Ingredients:

- 2 cups coconut milk
- 2 cup quinoa
- 8 eggs, whisked
- A pinch of black pepper
- 1 teaspoon turmeric powder
- 1 teaspoon chili powder
- 1 teaspoon rosemary, dried

Directions:

1. In your slow cooker, combine the milk with the quinoa, eggs and the other ingredients, put the lid on and cook on High for 2 hours.
2. Divide into bowls and serve for breakfast.

Nutrition Info:

Calories 720, Fat 42.7g, Cholesterol 327mg, Sodium 153mg, Carbohydrate 62.8g, Fiber 9.1g, Sugars 4.8g, Protein 26g, Potassium 942mg

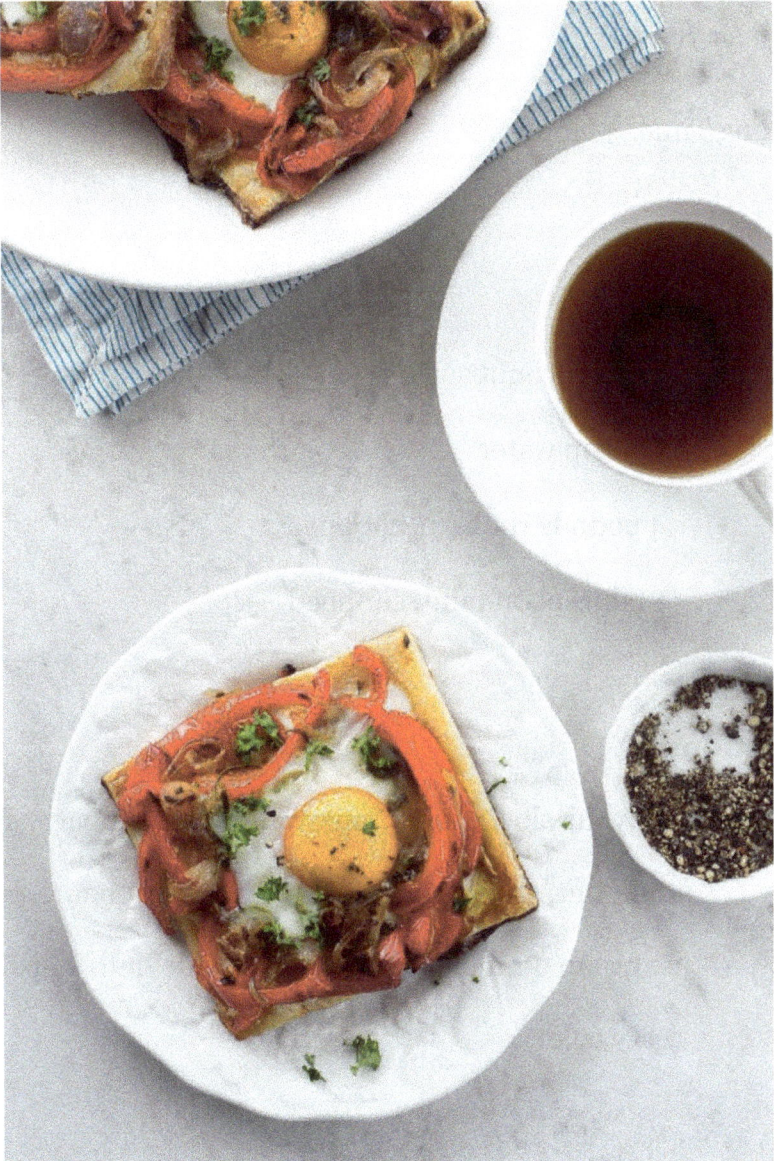

Rhubarb Dip

Servings: 8

Cooking Time: 3 Hours

Ingredients:

- 1 cup coconut sugar
- 1/3 cup water
- 4 pounds rhubarb, chopped
- 1 tablespoon mint, chopped

Directions:

1. In your slow cooker, mix water with rhubarb, sugar and mint, stir, cover, cook on High for 3 hours, blend using an immersion blender, divide into cups and serve cold.

Nutrition Info:

Calories 60, Fat 0.5g, Cholesterol 0mg, Sodium 15mg, Carbohydrate 12.7g, Fiber 4.1g, Sugars 2.5g, Protein 2.2g, Potassium 657mg

Honey Compote

Servings: 6

Cooking Time: 2 Hours

Ingredients:

- 64 ounces red grapefruit juice
- 1 cup honey
- ½ cup mint, chopped
- 1 cup water
- 2 grapefruits, peeled and chopped

Directions:

1. In your slow cooker, mix grapefruit with water, honey, mint and grapefruit juice, stir, cover, cook on High for 2 hours, divide into bowls and serve cold.

Nutrition Info:

Calories 364, Fat 0.1g, Cholesterol 0mg, Sodium 52mg, Carbohydrate 94.9g, Fiber 1.1g, Sugars 49.4g, Protein 0.7g, Potassium 124mg

Baby Spinach Shrimp Salad

Servings: 4

Cooking Time: 1 Hour

Ingredients:

- 1 pound shrimp, peeled and deveined
- 1 cup corn
- 1 cup baby spinach
- 1 cup cherry tomatoes, halved
- 1 teaspoon chili powder
- ½ cup low-sodium veggie stock
- 1 tablespoon cilantro, chopped

Directions:

1. In your slow cooker, combine the shrimp with the corn, spinach and the other ingredients, put the lid on and cook on High for 1 hour.
2. Divide into bowls and serve for breakfast.

Nutrition Info:

Calories 182, Fat .2.6g, Cholesterol 239mg, Sodium 346mg, Carbohydrate 11.9g, Fiber 2g, Sugars 2.6g, Protein 27.8g, Potassium 458mg

Cocoa Chia Pudding

Servings: 4

Cooking Time: 2 Hours

Ingredients:

- ½ cup coconut chia granola
- 2 tablespoons coconut, shredded and unsweetened
- 2 teaspoons cocoa powder
- ½ teaspoon vanilla extract
- ½ cup chia seeds
- 2 cups coconut milk
- ¼ cup maple syrup
- ½ teaspoon cinnamon powder

Directions:

1. In your slow cooker, mix chia granola with chia seeds, coconut milk, coconut, maple syrup, cinnamon, cocoa powder and vanilla, toss, cover and cook on High for 2 hours.
2. Divide chia pudding into bowls and serve for breakfast.

Nutrition Info: Calories 482, Fat 37.6g, Cholesterol 0mg, Sodium 32mg, Carbohydrate 32.5g, Fiber 11g, Sugars 17.5g, Protein 7.1g, Potassium 492mg

Apple Crisp

Servings: 5

Cooking Time: 4 Hrs 10 Mins

Ingredients:

- 1 cup Oatmeal
- 1 cup Brown Sugar
- 2 tbsp. Flour (all purpose)
- 1 tbsp. Sugar (granulated)
- 1 stick Butter
- 1 tsp. Cinnamon
- 1 lb. Apples (Granny Smith)

Directions:

1. Peel and thinly slice the apples.
2. Add flour and granulated sugar to the apples.
3. Coat them well.
4. Place them in the slow cooker.
5. Now, add remaining ingredients except oats.
6. Last, sprinkle the oatmeal on the apples.
7. Cook on "high" for 4 hrs.
8. Serve hot.

Nutrition Info:

(Estimated Amount Per Serving): 278 Calories; 10 g Total Fat; 134 mg Cholesterol; 270 mg Sodium; 8 mg Carbohydrates; 0 g Dietary Fiber; 32 g Protein

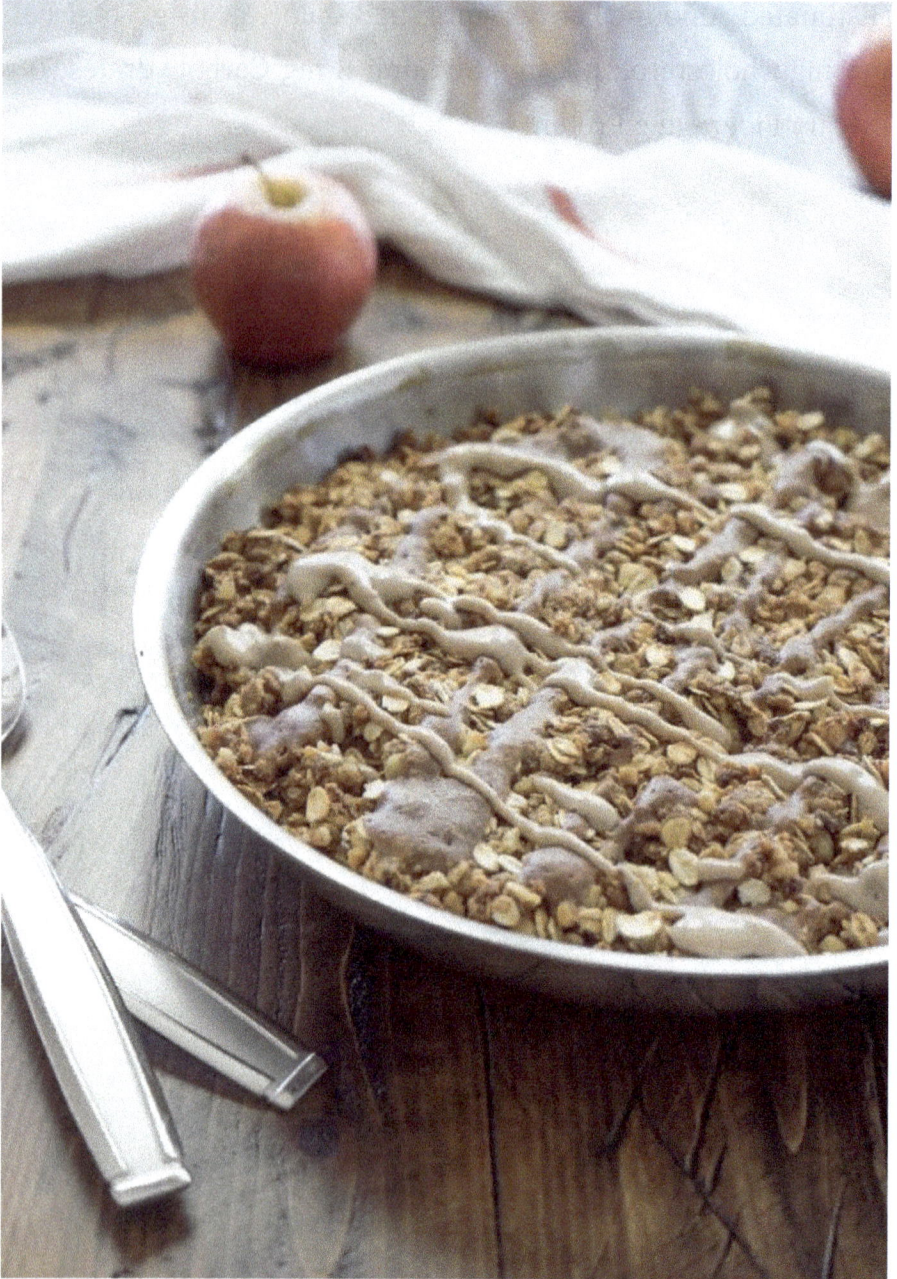

Coconut and Fruit Cake

Servings: 6

Cooking Time: 2 Hours And 30 Minutes

Ingredients:

- 1 cup mango, peeled and chopped
- 1 and ½ cups whole wheat flour
- ½ cup coconut milk
- 1 cup avocado, peeled, pitted and mashed
- ½ cup coconut flakes, unsweetened
- ½ teaspoon cinnamon powder

Directions:

1. In a bowl mix the mango with the flour and the other ingredients and whisk.
2. Line the slow cooker with parchment paper, pour the cake mix and cook on High fro 2 hours and 30 minutes.
3. Cool the cake down before slicing and serving it.

Nutrition Info:

Calories 249, Fat 12.2g, Cholesterol 0mg, Sodium 7mg, Carbohydrate 32.2g, Fiber 4g, Sugars 5g, Protein 4.6g, Potassium 274mg

Apple and Squash Bowls

Servings: 4

Cooking Time: 8 Hours

Ingredients:

- 1 teaspoon cinnamon powder
- ½ teaspoon nutmeg, ground
- ½ cup almonds
- ½ cup walnuts
- A splash of water
- 2 apples, peeled, cored and cubed
- 1 butternut squash, peeled and cubed
- 1 tablespoon stevia
- 1 cup coconut milk

Directions:

1. Put almonds and walnuts in your blender, add a splash of water, blend really well and transfer to your slow cooker.
2. Add apples, squash, cinnamon, stevia, nutmeg and coconut milk, stir, cover and cook on Low for 8 hours.
3. Stir, divide into bowls and serve.

Nutrition Info:

Calories 392, Fat 29.8g, Cholesterol 0mg, Sodium 19mg, Carbohydrate 30.5g, Fiber 7g, Sugars 19.8g, Protein 8.2g, Potassium 517mg

Slow Cooker Chocolate Cake

Servings: 8 Servings

Ingredients:

- 1¼ cups (285 g) brown sugar, divided
- 1 cup (125 g) flour
- ½ cup (45 g) unsweetened cocoa powder, divided
- 1½ teaspoons baking powder
- ½ cup (120 ml) skim milk
- 2 tablespoons (28 g) unsalted butter, melted
- ½ teaspoon vanilla
- 1¾ cups (410 ml) boiling water

Directions:

1. In a mixing bowl, mix together 1 cup (225 g) brown sugar, flour, ¼ cup (22 g) cocoa, and baking powder. Stir in milk, butter, and vanilla. Pour into slow cooker sprayed with nonstick cooking spray. In a separate bowl, mix together ¼ cup (60 g) brown sugar and ¼ cup (22 g) cocoa. Sprinkle over batter in the slow cooker. Do not stir. Pour boiling water over mixture. Do not stir. Cover and cook on high 1½ to 1¾ hours or until toothpick inserted into cake comes out clean.

Nutrition Info:

Per serving: 69 g water; 284 calories (11% from fat, 4% from protein, 84% from carb); 3 g protein; 4 g total fat; 2 g saturated fat; 1 g monounsaturated fat; 0 g polyunsaturated fat; 63 g carb; 2 g fiber; 46 g sugar; 104 mg phosphorus; 125 mg calcium; 2 mg iron; 123 mg sodium; 295 mg potassium; 120 IU vitamin A; 33 mg ATE vitamin E; 0 mg vitamin C; 8 mg cholesterol

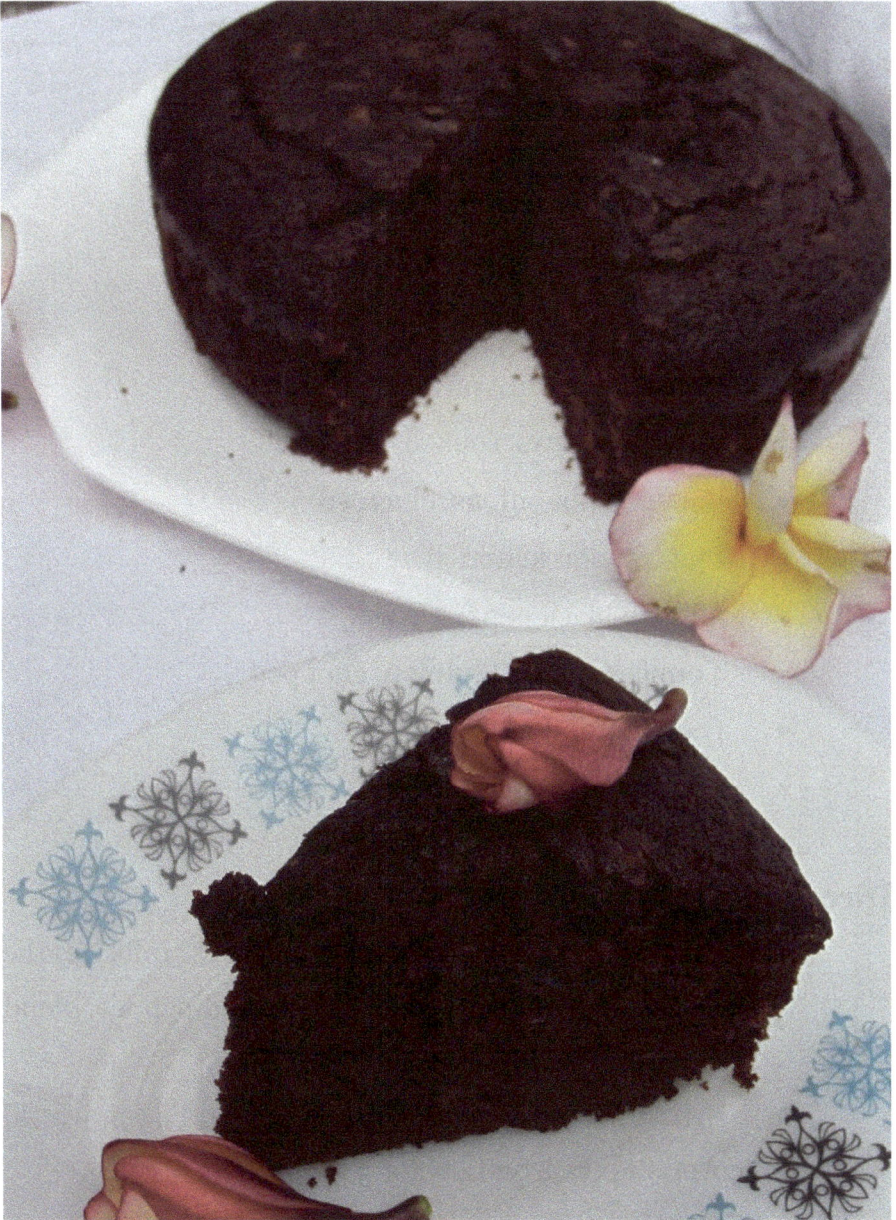

Fish Omelet

Servings: 3

Cooking Time: 3 Hours And 40 Minutes

Ingredients:

- 4 eggs, whisked
- ½ teaspoon olive oil
- ½ cup cashews, soaked, drained
- ¼ cup green onions, chopped
- 1 tablespoon lemon juice
- A pinch black pepper
- 4 ounces smoked salmon, chopped
- 1 cup almond milk
- 1 teaspoon garlic powder

Directions:

1. In your blender, mix cashews with milk, garlic powder, lemon juice, green onions and pepper, blend really well and leave aside.
2. Drizzle the oil in your slow cooker, add eggs, whisk, cover and cook on Low for 3 hours.

3. Add salmon, toss, cover, cook on Low for 40 minutes more, divide between plates, drizzle green onions sauce all over and serve.

Nutrition Info:

Calories 457, Fat 38g, Cholesterol 227mg, Sodium 856mg, Carbohydrate 13.8g, Fiber 2.8g, Sugars 4.8g, Protein 40g, Potassium 524mg

Brown Cake

Servings: 8

Cooking Time: 2 Hours And 30 Minutes

Ingredients:

- 1 cup flour
- 1 and ½ cup stevia
- ½ cup chocolate almond milk
- 2 teaspoons baking powder
- 1 and ½ cups hot water
- ¼ cup cocoa powder+ 2 tablespoons
- 2 tablespoons canola oil
- 1 teaspoon vanilla extract
- Cooking spray

Directions:

1. In a bowl, mix flour with ¼-cup cocoa, baking powder, almond milk, oil and vanilla extract, whisk well and spread on the bottom of the slow cooker greased with cooking spray.

2. In a separate bowl, mix stevia with the water and the rest of the cocoa, whisk well, spread over the batter,

cover, and cook your cake on High for 2 hours and 30 minutes.

3.   Leave the cake to cool down, slice and serve.

Nutrition Info:

Calories 150, Fat 7.6g, Cholesterol 1mg, Sodium 7mg, Carbohydrate 56.8g, Fiber 1.8g, Sugars 4.4g, Protein 2.9g, Potassium 185mg

Blueberries Cream

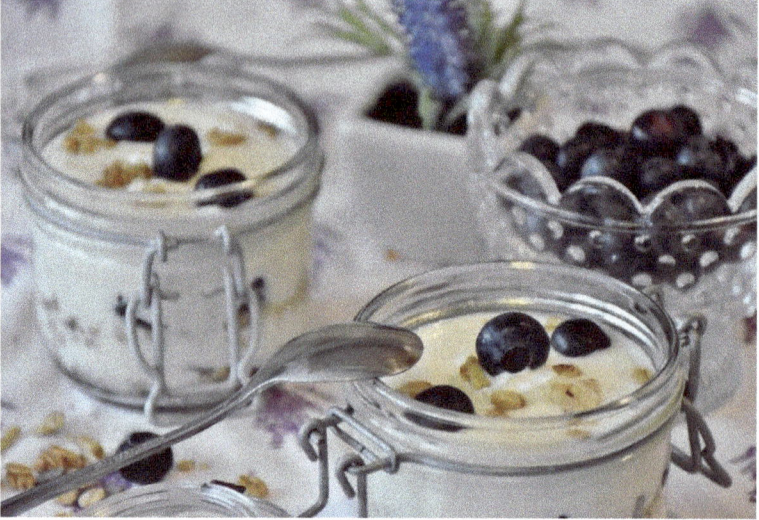

Servings: 10

Cooking Time: 1 Hour

Ingredients:

- 8 ounces mascarpone cheese
- 1 cup coconut cream
- 1 teaspoon stevia
- 1 pint blueberries

Directions:

1. In your slow cooker, mix the cream with stevia, mascarpone and the blueberries, stir, cover, cook on Low for 1 hour, divide bowls and serve cold.

Nutrition Info:

Calories 118, Fat 8.8g, Cholesterol 12mg, Sodium 23mg, Carbohydrate 8.4g, Fiber 1.5g, Sugars 4.9g, Protein 3.4g, Potassium 118mg

Stevia and Walnuts Cut Oats

Servings: 4

Cooking Time: 6 Hours

Ingredients:

- 1 tablespoon coconut oil
- 1 cup raspberries
- 4 tablespoons walnuts
- 2 cups water
- 1 cup nonfat milk
- 1 tablespoon stevia
- 1 cup steel cut oats
- ½ teaspoon vanilla extract

Directions:

1. In your slow cooker, combine the oil with the oats, water, milk, stevia, vanilla, raspberries and walnuts, cover and cook on Low for 6 hours.
2. Divide the oatmeal into bowls and serve.

Nutrition Info:

Calories 195, Fat 9.5g, Cholesterol 1mg, Sodium 38mg, Carbohydrate 28.9g, Fiber 4.6g, Sugars 4.7g, Protein 6.9g, Potassium 258mg

Spring Onions and Bacon Mix

Servings: 4

Cooking Time: 2 Hours And 30 Minutes

Ingredients:

- 8 eggs, whisked
- ½ cup low-sodium bacon, cooked and chopped
- ½ cup coconut cream
- 1 red bell pepper, chopped
- 2 spring onions, chopped
- ½ teaspoon chili powder
- A pinch of black pepper

Directions:

1. In the slow cooker, mix the eggs with the bacon, cream and the other ingredients, put the lid on and cook on High for 2 hours and 30 minutes.
2. Divide between plates and serve for breakfast.

Nutrition Info:

Calories 373, Fat 28.9g, Cholesterol 355mg, Sodium 390mg, Carbohydrate 5.3g, Fiber 1.4g, Sugars 3.4g, Protein 21.g, Potassium 280mg

Walnut and Cinnamon Oatmeal

Servings: 4

Cooking Time: 8 Hours

Ingredients:

- ½ cup gluten-free oats
- 1 carrot, grated
- ¼ teaspoon cloves, ground
- ¼ cup walnuts, chopped
- ½ teaspoon cinnamon powder
- 1 and ½ cups coconut milk
- ¼ zucchini, grated
- ¼ teaspoon nutmeg, ground
- 2 tablespoons stevia

Directions:

1. In your slow cooker, combine the oats with the carrot, zucchini, milk, nutmeg, cloves, cinnamon and stevia, cover and cook on Low for 8 hours.
2. Divide into bowls, sprinkle walnuts on top and serve.

Nutrition Info:

Calories 321, Fat .27.3g, Cholesterol 0mg, Sodium 26mg, Carbohydrate 25.5g, Fiber 5.3g, Sugars 4.1g, Protein 6.1g, Potassium 360mg

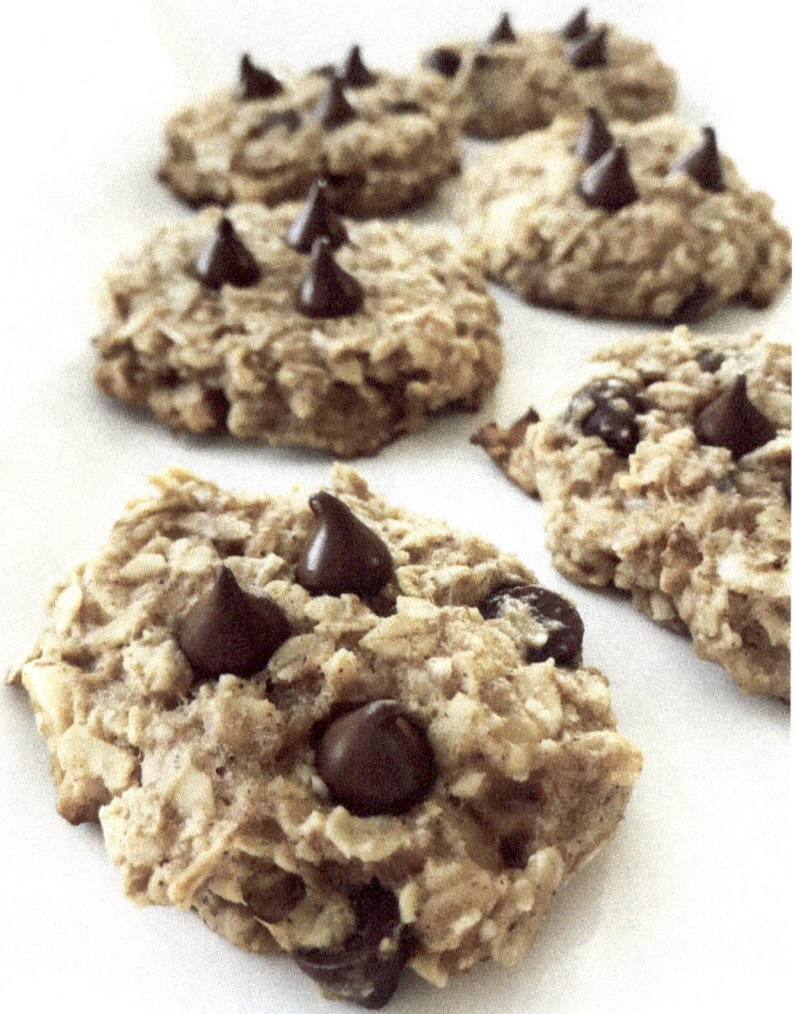

Pumpkin Pie Spices Cake

Servings: 6

Cooking Time: 2 Hours And 30 Minutes

Ingredients:

- 3 cups pears, cored and cubed
- 2 cups coconut flour
- 3 tablespoons stevia
- 2 eggs
- 1 tablespoon vanilla extract
- 1 tablespoon pumpkin pie spice
- 1 tablespoon baking powder
- 1 tablespoon avocado oil

Directions:

1. In a bowl mix eggs with the oil, spice, vanilla, pears and stevia and whisk well
2. In another bowl, mix baking powder with flour, stir, add to apples mix, stir again, transfer to your slow cooker, cover, cook on High for 2 hours and 30 minutes, slice and serve cold.

Nutrition Info:

Calories 22, Fat 6g, Cholesterol 55mg, Sodium 25mg, Carbohydrate 46.2g, Fiber 18.8g, Sugars 8.3g, Protein 7.6g, Potassium 382mg

Pears And Blackberries Bowls

Servings: 4

Cooking Time: 1 Hour

Ingredients:

- 1 cup apple, peeled, cored and cubed
- 1 cup blackberries
- 2 cups non-fat milk
- 2 tablespoons sugar
- ½ cup pears, peeled, cored and cubed
- ½ teaspoon vanilla extract

Directions:

1. In your slow cooker, combine the fruits with the milk and the other ingredients, put the lid on and cook on High for 1 hour.
2. Divide the mix into bowls and serve.

Nutrition Info:

Calories 125, Fat .0.3g, Cholesterol 2mg, Sodium 66mg, Carbohydrate 26.3g, Fiber 3.9g, Sugars 21.6g, Protein 4.7g, Potassium 332mg

Pears Mix

Servings: 6

Cooking Time: 1 Hour

Ingredients:

- 1 quart water
- 5 star anise
- 2 tablespoons stevia
- ½ pound pears, cored and cut into wedges
- ½ pound apple, cored and cut into wedges
- Zest of 1 orange, grated
- Zest of 1 lemon, grated
- 2 cinnamon sticks

Directions:

1. Put the water, stevia, apples, pears, star anise, and cinnamon, orange and lemon zest in your slow cooker, cover, cook on High for 1 hour, divide into bowls and serve cold.

Nutrition Info:

Calories 43, Fat 0.4g, Cholesterol 0mg, Sodium 6mg, Carbohydrate 14.3g, Fiber 2.7g, Sugars 5.9g, Protein 0.7g, Potassium 109mg

Tender Rosemary Sweet Potatoes

Servings: 8

Cooking Time: 7 Hour s

Ingredients:

- 1 tablespoon olive oil
- 2 tablespoons stevia
- 4 sweet potatoes, peeled and cut into wedges
- Black pepper to the taste
- ¼ cup water
- A pinch of rosemary, dried

Directions:

1. In your slow cooker, mix the potatoes with the oil, black pepper, rosemary, water and stevia, toss, cover and cook on Low for 7 hours.
2. Divide between plates and serve for breakfast.

Nutrition Info:

Calories 120, Fat 2.6g, Cholesterol 0mg, Sodium 147mg, Carbohydrate 26.8g, Fiber 3.2g, Sugars 1.5g, Protein 1.3g, Potassium 612mg

Orange and Maple Syrup Quinoa

Servings: 4

Cooking Time: 2 Hours

Ingredients:

- 1 cup quinoa
- 1 and ½ cups almond milk
- 1 orange, peeled and cut into segments
- 1 avocado, peeled, pitted and cubed
- 1 tablespoon maple syrup
- 1 teaspoon cinnamon powder
- ½ teaspoon almond extract

Directions:

1. In your slow cooker, combine the quinoa with the milk, orange and the other ingredients, put the lid on and cook on High for 2 hours.
2. Toss the mix, divide into bowls and serve.

Nutrition Info:

Calories 502, Fat 33.9g, Cholesterol 0mg, Sodium 19mg, Carbohydrate 45.4g, Fiber 9.4g, Sugars 10.6g, Protein 9.4g, Potassium 814mg

Vanilla and Nutmeg Oatmeal

Servings: 4

Cooking Time: 2 Hours

Ingredients:

- 1 cup old fashioned oats
- 2 cups non-fat milk
- 1 tablespoon sugar
- 1 teaspoon nutmeg, ground
- 1 teaspoon cinnamon powder
- 1 teaspoon vanilla extract

Directions:

1. In your slow cooker, combine the oats with the milk, nutmeg and the other ingredients, put the lid on and cook on High for 2 hours.
2. Divide the oatmeal into bowls and serve for breakfast.

Nutrition Info:

Calories 218, Fat 2.8g, Cholesterol 3mg, Sodium 65mg, Carbohydrate 36.7g, Fiber 4g, Sugars 10.4g, Protein 9g, Potassium 375mg

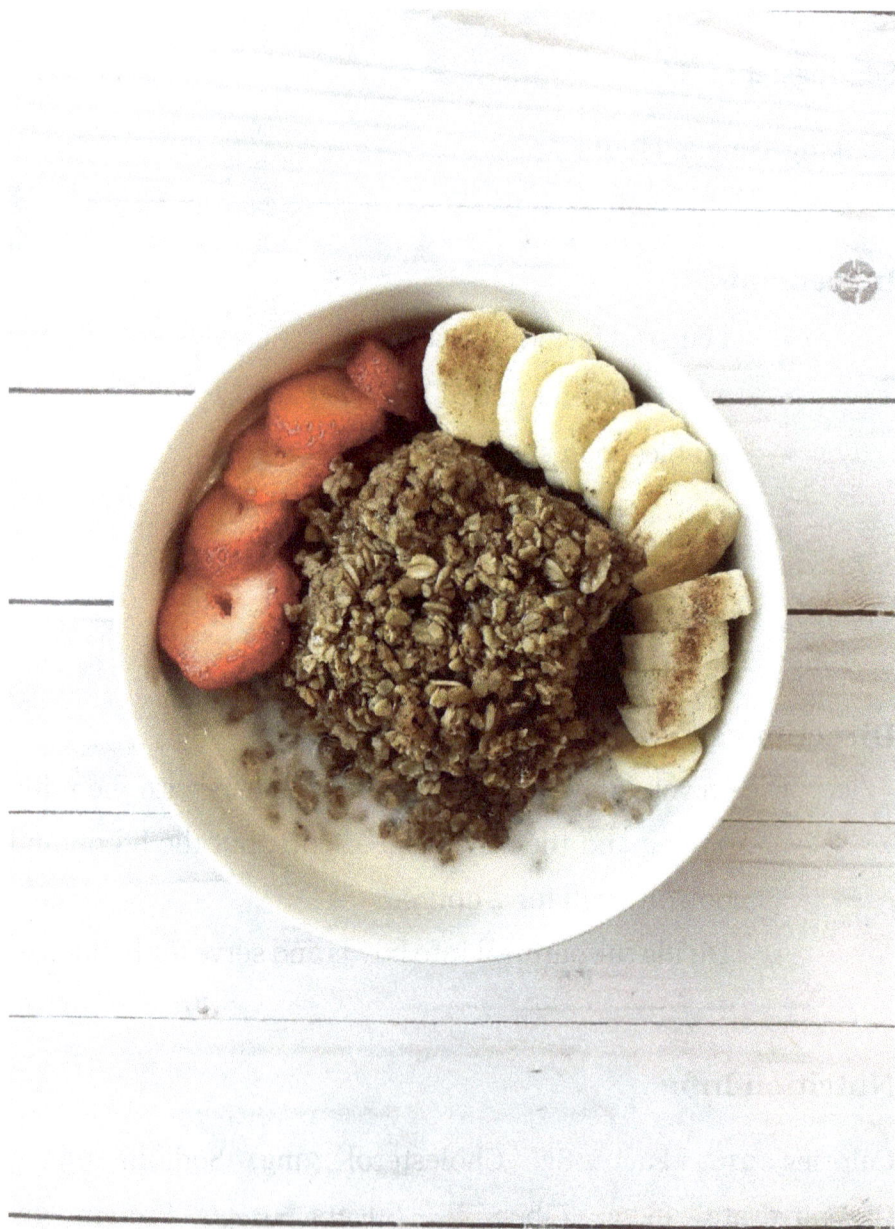

Pecans Cake

Servings: 4

Cooking Time: 5 Hours

Ingredients:

- Cooking spray
- 1 cup almond flour
- 1 cup orange juice
- 1 cup coconut sugar
- 3 tablespoons coconut oil, melted
- 1 teaspoon baking powder
- ½ teaspoon cinnamon powder
- ½ cup almond milk
- ½ cup pecans, chopped
- ¾ cup water
- ½ cup orange peel, grated

Directions:

1. In a bowl, mix flour with half of the sugar, baking powder, cinnamon, 2 tablespoons oil, milk and pecans, stir and pour this in your slow cooker greased with cooking spray.

2.   Heat up a small pan over medium heat, add water, orange juice, orange peel, the rest of the oil and the rest of the sugar, stir, bring to a boil, pour over the mix in the slow cooker, cover and cook on Low for 5 hours.

3.   Divide into bowls and serve cold.

Nutrition Info:

Calories 565, Fat 48.8g, Cholesterol 0mg, Sodium 28mg, Carbohydrate 26g, Fiber 7.8g, Sugars 7.1g, Protein 10.2g, Potassium 459mg

Stewed Apples

Servings: 6 Servings

Ingredients:

- 9 ounces (225 g) dried apples
- 1 cup (235 ml) orange juice
- 1 cup (235 ml) water
- ½ cup (120 ml) maple syrup
- 1 tablespoon (15 ml) lemon juice

Directions:

1. Place apples in slow cooker. Combine remaining ingredients and pour over apples. Cover and cook on low for 8 hours.

Nutrition Info:

Per serving: 124 g water; 109 calories (2% from fat, 2% from protein, 97% from carb); 0 g protein; 0 g total fat; 0 g saturated

fat; 0 g monounsaturated fat; 0 g polyunsaturated fat; 28 g carb;

1 g fiber; 20 g sugar; 10 mg phosphorus; 26 mg calcium; 0 mg

iron; 4 mg sodium; 175 mg potassium; 49 IU vitamin A; 0 mg ATE

vitamin E; 17 mg vitamin C; 0 mg cholesterol

Turmeric Hash Mix

Servings: 4

Cooking Time: 3 Hours

Ingredients:

- 1 pound hash browns
- 1 cup cherry tomatoes, halved
- 1 orange, peeled and cut into segments
- 1 tablespoon orange juice
- 1 and ½ teaspoon turmeric powder
- ½ cup low-sodium veggie stock
- A pinch of cayenne pepper

Directions:

1. In the slow cooker, combine the hash browns with the tomatoes, orange segments and the other ingredients, put the lid on and cook on High for 3 hours.
2. Divide into bowls and serve for breakfast.

Nutrition Info:

Calories 322, Fat .14.4g, Cholesterol omg, Sodium 439mg, Carbohydrate 44.7g, Fiber 4.4g, Sugars 4.8g, Protein 4g, Potassium 818mg

4-WEEK MEAL PLAN

Week 1

Monday
Breakfast: Tofu Frittata
Lunch: Pork Chops In Beer
Dinner: Stewed Tomatoes

Tuesday
Breakfast: Tapioca
Lunch: Creamy Beef Burgundy
Dinner: Oregano Salad

Wednesday
Breakfast: Fruit Oats
Lunch: Smothered Steak
Dinner: Black Beans With Corn Kernels

Thursday
Breakfast: Grapefruit Mix
Lunch: Pork For Sandwiches
Dinner: Stuffed Acorn Squash

Friday
Breakfast: Berry Yogurt
Lunch: Cranberry Pork Roast

Dinner: Greek Eggplant

Saturday
Breakfast: Soft Pudding
Lunch: Pan-asian Pot Roast
Dinner: Thyme Sweet Potatoes

Sunday
Breakfast: Black Beans Salad
Lunch: Short Ribs
Dinner: Barley Vegetable Soup

Week 2

Monday
Breakfast: Carrot Pudding
Lunch: French Dip
Dinner: Butter Corn

Tuesday
Breakfast: Apple Cake
Lunch: Italian Roast With Vegetables
Dinner: Orange Glazed Carrots

Wednesday
Breakfast: Almond Milk Barley Cereals
Lunch: Honey Mustard Ribs
Dinner: Cinnamon Acorn Squash

Thursday

Breakfast: Cashews Cake

Lunch: Pizza Casserole

Dinner: Glazed Root Vegetables

Friday

Breakfast: Artichoke Frittata

Lunch: Hawaiian Pork Roast

Dinner: Stir Fried Steak, Shiitake And Asparagus

Saturday

Breakfast: Mexican Eggs

Lunch: Apple Cranberry Pork Roast

Dinner: Cilantro Brussel Sprouts

Sunday

Breakfast: Stewed Peach

Lunch: Swiss Steak

Dinner: Italian Zucchini

Week 3

Monday

Breakfast: Lamb Cassoule t

Lunch: Glazed Pork Roast

Dinner: Cilantro Parsnip Chunks

Tuesday

Breakfast: Fruited Tapioca

Lunch: Swiss Steak In Wine Sauce

Dinner: Corn Casserole

Wednesday

Breakfast: Baby Spinach Shrimp Salad

Lunch: Italian Pork Chops

Dinner: Pilaf With Bella Mushrooms

Thursday

Breakfast: Coconut And Fruit Cake

Lunch: Italian Pot Roast

Dinner: Italian Style Yellow Squash

Friday

Breakfast: Apple And Squash Bowls

Lunch: Beef With Horseradish Sauce

Dinner: Stevia Peas With Marjoram

Saturday

Breakfast: Slow Cooker Chocolate Cake

Lunch: Oriental Pot Roast

Dinner: Broccoli Rice Casserole

Sunday

Breakfast: Fish Omelet

Lunch: Barbecued Ribs

Dinner: Italians Style Mushroom Mix

Week 4

Monday
Breakfast: Brown Cake
Lunch: Ham And Scalloped Pota toes
Dinner: Broccoli Casserole

Tuesday
Breakfast: Stevia And Walnuts Cut Oats
Lunch: Pork And Pineapple Roast

Wednesday
Breakfast: Walnut And Cinnamon Oatmeal
Lunch: Barbecued Brisket
Dinner: Dinner: Slow Cooker Lasagna

Thursday
Breakfast: Tender Rosemary Sweet Potatoes
Lunch: Barbecued Short Ribs
Dinner: Brussels Sprouts Casserole

Friday
Breakfast: Orange And Maple Syrup Quinoa
Lunch: Beer-braised Short Ribs
Dinner: Pasta And Mushrooms

Saturday
Breakfast: Vanilla And Nutmeg Oatmeal
Lunch: Lamb Stew
Dinner: Onion Cabbage

Sunday

Breakfast: Pecans Cake

Lunch: Barbecued Ham

Dinner: Cheese Broccoli

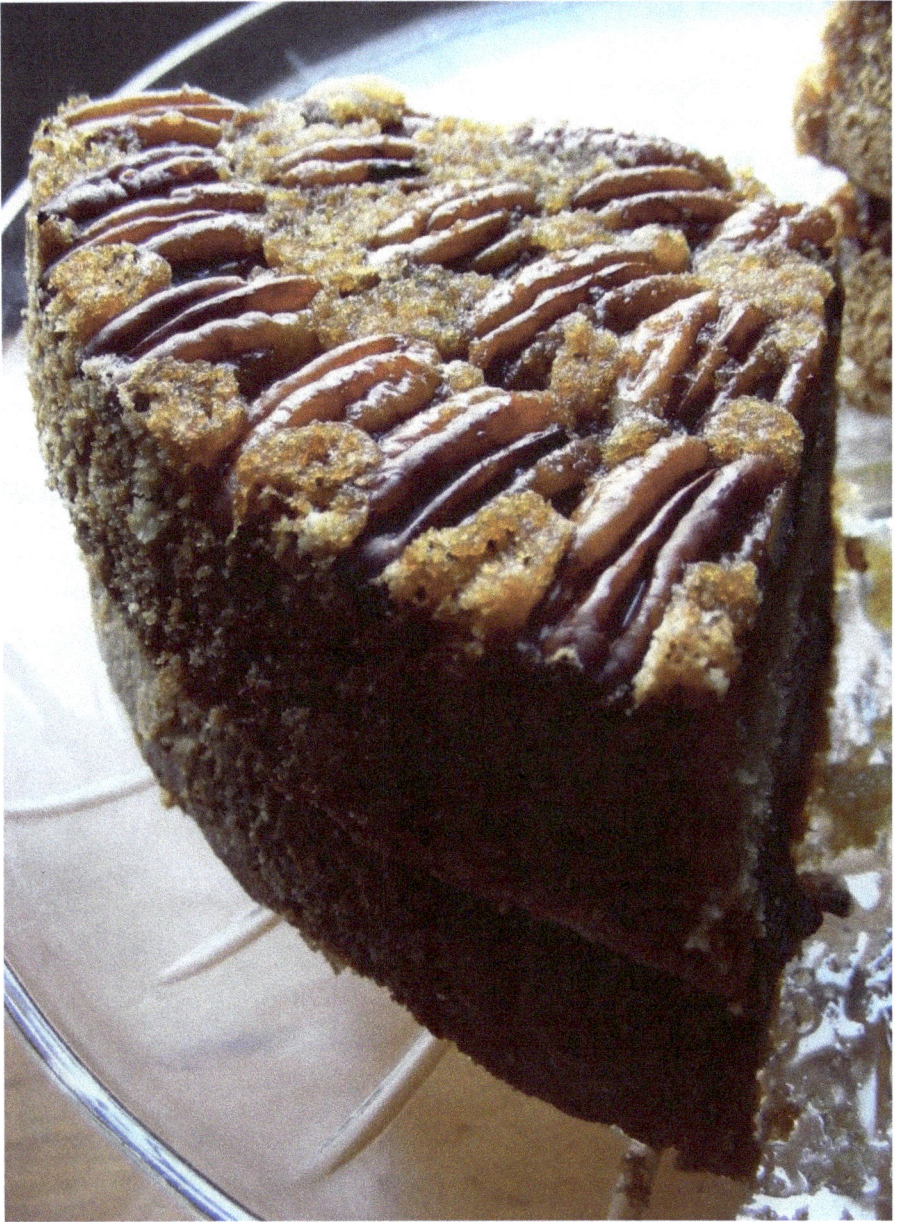

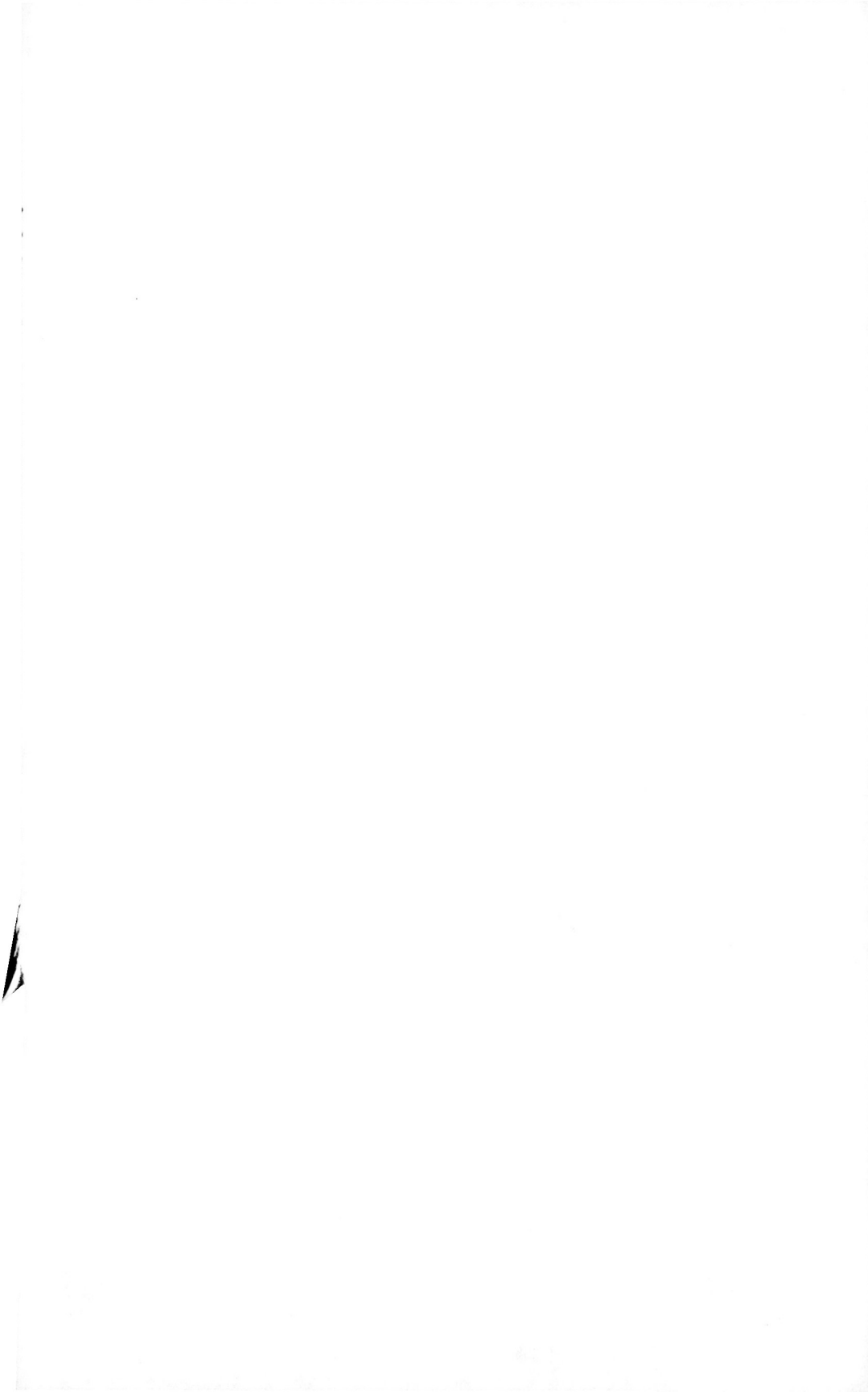

www.ingramcontent.com/pod-product-compliance
Lightning Source LLC
Chambersburg PA
CBHW050217270326
41914CB00003BA/453